© 2015 by Stacey Carson

HOW TO FEEL AND LOOK YOUNGER

By Stacey Carson

Disclaimer.

The author of this book does not dispense medical advice or prescribe the use of any technique as a form of treatment for physical, emotional, or medical problems without the advice of a physician, either directly or indirectly.
The intent of the author is only to offer information of a general nature to help you in your quest for emotional and spiritual well-being.
In the event you use any of the information in this book for yourself, which is your constitutional right, the author and the publisher assume no responsibility for your actions.

Even though the author has practiced all of the exercises in this book and believes that she has benefited from doing them, that has not been scientifically proven and it also neither means nor implies that you would experience similar results or success. Basically, you should always seek the opinion of a medical professional before you undertake any exercise program.

Dedication

Firstly, I would like thank A. V. Demenshin and M.S. Norbekov, whose trainings provided the basis for much of what is contained herein.

I took their basic trainings and adapted them for my purposes.

What is in this book is what I have found worked for me and I hope it will work for you, if you choose to apply it.

I would like to thank my daughter, her husband, my granddaughters, my son, his wife, and my grandson.

And, most importantly, Joseph Masiokas without whose help and encouragement this book would not exist.

© 2015 by Stacey Carson

Table of Contents

Introduction

This book examines how energy, humor, specific exercises (both physical and mental), and breathing can rejuvenate and cleanse the human body.

Good humor and laughter work wonders in the body. They destroy negative emotions, act as a tonic or medicine, cure certain ailments, and give new power.

The spirit of laughter is of great importance to our lives and will be examined in some detail. Certain body rejuvenation exercises are presented herein.

The importance of the spine to the quality of our life is discussed and exercises to help straighten the spine so that our life can be filled with more joy are detailed.

Quite a few of the exercises described rely on the power of one's thoughts and imagination. Vividly imagining cleansing certain parts of the body, like the intestines, liver, and kidneys, can help improve our overall health and the joy we receive from living.

Controlled breathing is important to the performance of many of the exercises contained herein as well as to the relaxation of our eyes, when they are tired or strained from working.

And being able to exhale the stale air inside of our lungs and replace it with fresh air works wonders.

By becoming more positive and taking charge of our bodies, we can change our emotions and our control over the health of our bodies.

It will take time, effort, and desire to realize the results that are mentioned in the book, but it can be very physically, emotionally, and spiritually rewarding.

The author has been very happy with her progress and the fact that most people think she is at least fifteen years younger than her chronological age.

The author discovered most of the exercises and activities proposed in this book by studying traditional medicine and less traditional medicine from the East; although the author chose things that worked for her and, in many instances, modified the teachings of those she studied to arrive at exercises and practices that she felt were more personally beneficial for herself. She is so happy with her own progress that she chose to share her program with others so that they may benefit as she has done.

While she cannot offer any particular guarantees that others will be as successful with this program as she has been, she would like others to begin thinking about what they can do to take charge of their health, their vitality, their joy and their spirit.

Good health and good humor to you.

1. Energy

1.1. Body position and movement.

You cannot purchase a good mood, you need to create your good mood yourself. If your brain is overloaded with information, take a break, go for a walk, or meditate.

Scientists have long ago discovered that anxiety and anger directly destroy internal organs, but it is equally known that there is an inverse relationship: a healthy attitude fills us with a sense of strength, dance purifies the mind blocks created while sitting tense and cross-legged (and therefore less able to breathe fully), ends vulnerability and fearful emotions, not to mention that eerie feeling inside that something is wrong. Body position and movement changes the state of consciousness.

1. 2. Attention and emotion.

Fear, anger, anxiety, jealousy, pain are oscillating at low frequencies. Love, joy, compassion vibrate at high frequencies.

If you have no energy, then you are in a bad mood. A person is then is upset, mad, and life is just not interesting anymore. The person then only wants to sleep all day and do nothing at all. If someone is full of energy, then they want to do everything they can. They want to laugh and are awake all day. They feel like they have a life that is full of excitement.

Man easily takes on the surrounding emotions and sentiments, often without even realizing how this changes his wellness.

Mood affects different areas of our life: marriage, work, self-confidence, and even satisfaction with life in general.

Recent studies suggest that a good mood is caught as fast as a bad one. Probably because we like to be among happy people--their mood quickly spills over to us.

One's prevailing mood at work is a combination of the atmosphere at home and work performance. Research shows that well-minded people work more productively and efficiently than their irritable colleagues.

1. 3. Your energy is impacted by what you are thinking about.

What you think about has an impact on your mental condition and your wellness. If you are thinking about the problems at work, your mind and body are being debilitated by the negative properties associated with this. Experience something new, perhaps take a look at something blue in color.

Different colors cause different emotions, and blue is the color of relaxation and tranquility. Studies have shown that touches -- be it from a massage or stroking a dog, or just holding hands with a spouse or lover-- helps reduce blood pressure, improves resistance to stress and overall mood and energy.

When we say, "Oh, he got out of bed on the wrong side", we mean that the person does not feel smart and happy, maybe he thinks that nobody can change his mood.

But our moods are shaped by our thoughts, which we choose -- so it is definitely possible to change a bad mood into a good mood.

And finally, if you're feeling sad, try to smile, no matter how badly you feel. Your mood will change eventually, and your relationship with others improves.

1.4. Energy charge.

When you wake up in the morning, you need to charge your energy. There is a simple way of doing that.

Lying in bed you put your hand under your head on the neck at the point where the hair begins to grow. Inhale deeply as far as you can and exhale as slowly as you can. Do this for 10-15 minutes. You will feel like the energy flowing into your body.

Put a smile on your face.

2. Laughter

More recently, scientists have begun to explain why we laugh. Why do we have to open our mouths and make those strange sounds? Why it is fun to laugh? How and why it works in our body? Of course, they have discovered that every 10-minute attack of laughter prolongs our life itself.

Laughter produces vitamin C. 10 seconds of delicious laughter from the belly can raise heart rate to the level reached after 10 minutes of rowing. Studies have shown that after 10 minutes of laughing, the laughing activated white cells in our blood that are responsible for infectious virus detection and elimination of those viruses.

Funny people tend to be healthier, because, as you know, laughing improves the physical condition and determines the state of consciousness. Laughter relaxes the body and is an important weapon in the fight against stress – over time; laughter slows the heart rate and lowers blood pressure.

Laughter inhibits stress in the body and most importantly - human laughter reduces anger - a key condition for getting heart attacks. Smile and the world smiles with you. It's not only a beautiful thought, but also studies confirm it to be true.

Most human problems are related to existing internal constraints and tensions. The consequences of these internal constraints are various diseases, various complexes, and fear. All of these conditions do not allow a person to enjoy life.

2.1. Laughter is the key to looking younger

The more you laugh the younger you will look. Most adults only smile 15 or less times per day. Smiling, itself, will perform miracles—it will make your immune system stronger, it will reduce production of your stress hormone, it will reduce the levels of pain you feel, it will eliminate many microbes from your body, and it will reduce the likelihood of having a stroke or heart attack. All of these positive effects and

you do not even have to pay for any medicines--
because laughter is for free.

If you spend 40 minutes in deep relaxation, a
state similar to meditation, you will produce the
same results in your body as 10 minute of honest
smiling. If you have any problem and you can
look at the situation with humor, you will find it
much easier to solve.

Laughing heartily for ten minutes will produce
the same effect in your body as two hours of
very deep sleep. Two to three minutes of intense
laughing to the point of producing tears in your
eyes, will relax your body better than anything
else can.

Laughing for ten minutes produces more
positive results for your body than forty minutes
of exercise will. It could be considered
respiratory gymnastics.
Ha ha is from your heart.
He he is from your third eye
Ho ho is from your diaphragm.

We inhale more air than we exhale and then our
lungs become dirty, so laughter helps to clean
the lungs because we push more air out of them.

Deep laughter makes us cough which helps to clean our airway. Once again, laughing is like medicine—but for **FREE!**

Your brain cannot tell the difference between you laughing because you find something humorous or you laughing because you want to laugh for the positive effects of laughter on your body. Try, try, try to laugh without any particular reason every day and it will make you feel better. If you find that embarrassing, you can laugh in private, by yourself. One of the most effective ways of improving your mood and your wellness--laughter therapy! Large internal constraints and tensions may be removed by sincerely laughing.

Everyone knows that laughter and good humor have a strong impact on treating illnesses. This was proven by Norman Cousins in the early 1970s. However, to achieve the maximum effects of laughter therapy, laughter must be applied correctly and in moderation. Sigmund Freud argued that the circumstances corresponding to laughter can reduce the chances of conflicts. Smiling strengthens the body's immune system. Laughter is remarkable in that it is a human **REFLEX**, the only human characteristic psychological act, in which our subconscious mind, and body are participants.

As a reflex it can detect when it is exposed to sensitive parts of the body - for example being tickled under the arm can cause laughter as can losing one's swim suit when leaving a stormy sea

How does laughter work: the brain increases calming and analgesic substances – endorphins, spasmodic movements of the ribs and shaking them around existing muscle groups (hence the expression laughing until it hurts), and the lungs work intensively to displace large volumes of air.

Vision becomes sharper due to increased number of tears in the eyes--this is the emergence of reflex tears, which result in a smile.

When you smile your face muscles tighten and your nostrils dilate.

3. The exercise: rejuvenating the body

Former British Army Colonel Bradford (a pscudonym) was almost 70-years old and wanted to feel young again. He went to the Himalayan Mountains in search of the secret to eternal youth.

He found a group of Tibetan monks who told him the secret of eternal youth passed down from generation to generation. They told him of old men who inexplicably became healthy, strong, and full of vigor.

Former colonel Bradford stayed with the monks for several years. His outward appearance became younger—some said he looked almost 40 years younger. His friends did not recognize Bradford. He became an erect, dark-haired, fresh-faced man.

What the monks told former Colonel Bradford about were five Tibetan body exercises. They work on stiff muscles and joints and tighten muscles. They help regulate the body's functions and inhibit aging. In addition to the exercises they gave him other principles to live by, like eliminating alcohol.

We know that the muscles weaken with age. We also know that beautiful posture will produce pride in our posture and bearing. While doing the following exercises put a smile on your face and imagine that you only eighteen—young and limber. Mentally remind your brain that you are healthy, strong, and happy. Success accompanies you day and night. You must put yourself into what you think. With each repetition inspire yourself to produce a positive feature

For the first week, perform the exercise 3 times.
The second week do it 5 times.
On the third week perform it 7 times.
On the fourth week perform it 9 times.
On the fifth week perform it 11 times.
In the sixth week, do it 13 times.
The seventh week 15 times.
The eighth week, do it 17 times.
The ninth week perform it19 times.
In the tenth week and beyond perform it 21 times.

3.1. The first position.

Rotate your entire body clockwise three times. Arms are extended to the sides with palms down. When you have finished spinning, you have to stand for a few seconds. Your hands should then be placed in a position of prayer. The exercise is repeated 3 times and each week you add 2 repetitions until you reach 21.

3. 2. The second position.

You lie down on your back with your legs stretched out.

Feet pressed close to each other, foot upright. Your hands are next to your buttocks, palms facing down.

At the same time, lift your legs and head up. Strain for your chin to touch your chest. Raising your legs to the top, stretched out over your knees. Try to lower your feet to touch the floor near your head. Do not force yourself to stretch too far; only go as far as you can go easily.
After that, slowly lower your legs and head. Relax your muscles.

Each time you raise your legs and head take in a deep breath, and when lowering your legs and head slowly and deeply exhale.
You perform this exercise 3 times the first week and add 2 repetitions each week thereafter.

When you have completed your repetitions, lie down on your back and stretch your arms to the sides, palms up, for a couple of minutes.

3.3. The third position.

Kneel on the floor. Legs apart. Your back and head straight, arms are extended and resting on the buttocks.

Take a deep breath. Bend your head down attempting to touch your chin to your chest.

Long deep exhalation as you return your head up and then bending it backwards. Your spine will be curved backwards but will be supported by your hands on the posterior part of the hip.

Take a deep breath with your head back and exhale it as you return your head to an upright position.

The exercise is repeated 3 times; and each week you add 2 repetitions until you reach 21.
At the end of the third position repetitions, remain kneeling on the floor and let your body and head fall forward and rest it on the floor for

a couple of minutes before moving on to the fourth position.

3. 4. The fourth position.

Sit down on the floor with your legs outstretched in front of you and your feet together with your toes pointed upward. The back is straight and the palms of your hands are on the floor next to you. Then spread your legs with bent knees and feet on the floor comfortably apart. Your arms are now behind your body with the palms on the floor. Palms and toes are both in a forward position on the floor.

Your body is pushed off of the floor and you press your chin towards your chest. Then recline your head as far as possible and raise your waist.

Knees bent and hands outstretched. Shins are perpendicular. Your back is parallel to the floor. Take a deep breath when your back is raised and hold it until you are on the way back to the starting position.

After the exercise repetitions are finished, sit a couple of minutes on the floor. The first week perform 3 repetitions and increase the number of repetitions by 2 each week until you have reached 21.

3. 5. Fifth position.

Face the floor and get down on your hands and knees, in a sort of push up position. Move into a position with your back in a bow over the floor, supported by your hand and feet and your butt is at the apex of height. Then bend your head back as far as possible and lower your body without touching the floor.

Breathe deeply as you are raising your body up and exhale when you are returning to the starting position.

After you have completed your repetitions, which are only 3 the first week, rest for a couple of minutes on your knees, allowing your head to fall forward onto the floor, either with your hands stretched out in front of your body or with them resting back past your knees.
For the first week you perform 3 repetitions and every week add two repetitions until you have reached 21.

4. Spine stretching

Posture stimulates your brain, so it is a great tool for overcoming depression. It is impossible to fall into a depression if the posture is straight, head raised high, deep breathing, and lips showing a smile!

While doing this exercise keep on a SMILE on your face! Correct posture helps: maintain good health, act directly on our emotions, strengthen the abdominal muscles, strengthen the body's energy centers, maintain a good mood, and prevent depression.

The spine is extremely important and critical to everyone's physical health! Our body structure is perfectly appropriate. The human skeleton with muscles is accurately adjusted leverage -- very simple and universal. If you want to recover from any illness, the spine should be straight.

Ivan P. Pavlov has proven, many years ago, that humans and animals can develop conditioned reflexes.

Applying Pavlov's discovery, if we perform stretching exercises for the spine 40 times, the spine will automatically stretch out without our conscious effort.

When you have done this exercise forty separate times, your body will automatically keep your spine straighter and you will have improved posture. A straight spine solves a lot of health problems. Bending the spine compresses the organs and this causes health problems.

Make an exercise out of imagining what it is you seek in your life. The most effective way to do it is while sitting on a hard chair in a warm room. Place your palms on your thighs. This will strengthen the natural rise of your lungs and will intensify your thoughts.

Imagination -- enables us to become what we want. Just imagine in great detail is what you seek.

4. 1. While sitting on a hard chair in a warm room, imagine, as a stream of warm water rises from the coccyx toward the waist, upper back, shoulders, and up to the upper part of the neck where the hair starts. Stretch your spine as much as possible as it is traveling upwards.

The spine should remain straight while the stream of warm water drops back to your coccyx.

4. 2. And again, imagine, as a stream of warm water rises from the coccyx toward the waist, upper back, shoulders, and up to the upper part of the neck where the hair starts. Stretch your spine as much as possible as it is traveling upwards.

The spine should remain straight while the stream of warm water drops back to your coccyx.

4. 3. And once again, imagine, as a stream of warm water rises from the coccyx toward the waist, upper back, shoulders, and up to the upper part of the neck where the hair starts. Stretch your spine as much as possible as it is traveling upwards.

The spine should remain straight while the stream of warm water drops back to your coccyx.

4. 4. Imagine, as a stream of warm water rises from the coccyx moving in a sine wave pattern from left to right vertically rising to the waist, upper back, shoulders, and up to the upper part of the neck where the hair line starts.

Stretch your spine even further this time than before if at all possible.

The spine should remain straight while the stream of warm water drops back to your coccyx.

4. 5. Imagine again this stream of warm water rising from the coccyx moving in a sine wave pattern from back to front vertically, raising to the waist, upper back, shoulders, and up to the upper part of the neck where the hair starts. Attempt to stretch the spine even more that previously.

Stretch your spine as high as you can with each upward movement. Massaging the spine like this improves blood circulation.

The spine should remain straight while the stream of warm water drops back to your coccyx.

4. 6. Imagine, as a stream of warm water rises circling around the spine in a clockwise rotation from the coccyx toward the waist, upper back, shoulders, and up to the upper part of the neck where the hair starts. Stretch your spine as much as possible as it is traveling upwards.

The spine should remain straight while the stream of warm water recedes in a bigger counterclockwise rotation circling around the spine to the coccyx.

4. 7. Imagine, as a stream of warm water rises circling around the spine in counterclockwise rotation from the coccyx toward the waist, upper back, shoulders, and up to the upper part of the neck where the hair starts. Stretch your spine as much as possible as the warm water is traveling upwards.

The spine should remain straight while the stream of warm water recedes in a bigger clockwise rotation circling around the spine to the coccyx.

After this exercise relax your body and sit for one minute.

After a minute imagine that it is a hot summer day and you are in the refreshing room. Cool refreshing air refreshes your body.

4. 8. Imagine, as a stream of cool water rises from the coccyx toward the waist, upper back, shoulders, and up to the upper part of the neck where the hair starts. Stretch your spine as much as possible as the water is traveling upwards.

The spine should remain straight while the stream of cool water drops back to your coccyx.

4. 9. And again, imagine, as a stream of cool water rises from the coccyx toward the waist, upper back, shoulders, and up to the upper part of the neck where the hair starts. Stretch your spine as much as possible as the cool water is traveling upwards.

The spine should remain straight while the stream of cool water drops back to your coccyx.

4. 10. And once again, imagine a stream of cool water rising from the coccyx toward the waist, upper back, shoulders, and up to the upper part of the neck where the hair starts. Stretch your spine as much as possible as it is traveling upwards.

The spine should remain straight while the stream of cool water drops back to your coccyx.

4. 11. Imagine, as a stream of cool water rises from the coccyx, moving in a sine wave pattern from left to right vertically, to the waist, upper back, shoulders, and to the upper part of the neck where the hair line starts. Stretch your spine even further this time than before, if at all possible.

The spine should remain straight while the stream of cool water drops back to your coccyx.

4. 12. Imagine again this stream of cool water rising from the coccyx moving in a sine wave pattern from back to front vertically to the waist, upper back, shoulders, and up to the upper part of the neck where the hair starts. Attempt to stretch the spine even more than previously.

Stretch your spine as high as you can with each upward movement. Massaging the spine like this improves blood circulation.

The spine should remain straight while the stream of cool water drops back to your coccyx.

4. 13. Imagine, as a stream of cool water rises circling around the spine in a clockwise rotation from the coccyx toward the waist, upper back, shoulders, and up to the upper part of the neck where the hair starts. Stretch your spine as much as possible as the cool water is traveling upwards.

The spine should remain straight while the stream of cool water recedes in a bigger counterclockwise rotation circling around the spine to the coccyx.

Imagine as a stream of cool water rises circling around the spine in counterclockwise rotation from the coccyx toward the waist, upper back, shoulders, and up to the upper part of the neck where the hair starts. Stretch your spine as much as possible as it is traveling upwards

The spine should remain straight while the stream of cool water recedes in a bigger clockwise rotation circling around the spine to the coccyx.

After this exercise relax your body and sit for one minute.

If you realize the importance of body posture, you begin to consciously pay attention to the position of the body!

Dear friends, who are reading these thoughts, lie back and think of life on its axis -- the spine!
A straight spine and erect posture slows the aging rate!
Straightening the spine can overcome a bad mood and tiredness!

5. Making Your Organs Younger

Speaking of the subconscious mind and the imagination and how they can affect one's life, take for example the life story of Dr. Milton H. Erickson.

Dr. Erickson was born with a variety of problems: color blindness, dyslexia, difficulty distinguishing '3' and 'm', tone deafness, and pollen allergy so severe that it required hospitalization from time to time. The combination of those would not be considered so very overwhelming, but when he was 17, he contracted poliomyelitis and it was such a devastating form of the disease that three doctors told his parents he would not live to see the next day's sunset. Milton overheard that and determined that he would live.

5. 1. Intestine Cleaning.

As we age our internal organs, like the small intestine, become less efficient. The intestinal villi—part of the small intestine involved with absorbing nutrients from consumed food— become less effective. If a child eats an apple, their intestine will grab more vitamins than if an adult were to eat an apple. In order for an aging or aged body to metabolize nutrients more efficiently drinking water cleans the intestine and the bowel.

After cleaning the intestine, the absorption of nutrients is greater, and the skin become cleaner, more moisturized, and fresher. You also get strengthened immunity. Science says this about the strength of immunity--the older you are, the smaller the amount of vitamins you will get from your food. So it is good to clean the intestine.

You should love yourself, spoil your body. Only you can spoil yourself better than anybody else can.
What should you do for cleaning your intestine? IMAGINE that you are walking down a corridor toward the most beautiful door you have ever seen. You open the door an IMAGINE that you walk into a nice, cozy, warm room. When you get there, you take off your clothing and you go to sit on chair in the middle of the room.

You then IMAGINE that warm water flows through the right-hand side of your abdomen and bottom like a jar would fill the abdominal cavity

with water. Your hand touches the lower part of the abdomen on the right side.
You move your hand in a clockwise motion toward the solar ring. You keep going in a circle to the left side of the abdomen.

Then, go in the same motion two more times. After making three larger circles, you keep going but in a smaller circle three times. Then, go in the same motion but make the circle larger three times.

When you have completed nine circles, you realize that you have washed your intestines.

Gather the weightless turbid water in the lower abdomen. This dirty water is allowed to flow into a container located on the ground next to your right-hand side. Your clean intestines glow with all the colors of the rainbow.

Again you IMAGINE that warm water flows through the right-hand side of the abdomen and bottom like a jar would fill the abdominal cavity with water. Your hand touches the lower part of the abdomen on the right side.

You move your hand in a clockwise motion

toward the solar ring. You keep going in a circle to the left side of the abdomen.

Then, go in the same motion two more times. After making three larger circles, you keep going but in a smaller circle three times. Then, go in the same motion but make the circle larger three times.

When you have completed nine circles, you realize that you have washed your intestines.

Gather the weightless turbid water in the lower abdomen. This dirty water is allowed to flow into a container located on the ground next to your right-hand side. Your clean intestines glow more brilliantly with all the colors of the rainbow.

Now use lukewarm water.

You IMAGINE that lukewarm water flows through the right-hand side of the abdomen and bottom like a jar filling the abdominal cavity with water.

Again your hand touches the lower part of the abdomen on the right side. You move your hand in a clockwise motion toward the solar ring.

You keep going in a circle to the left side of the abdomen. Then, go in the same motion two more times. You keep going in a smaller circle and keep making the motion three times.

Then, go in the same motion but make the circle larger three times. Rotate the hand and touching your belly, you realize that you have washed your intestines.

Gather the clean water in the lower abdomen. Your clean water is allowed to flow into a container located on the ground next to your right-hand side. Your intestines light up three times more vividly in all the colors of the rainbow.
Follow this exercise by sitting for a couple of minutes so that your brain can consider what you have done.

After this procedure, your intestine will clean itself over the next 2-3 days.

Repeat this procedure in the spring and autumn, or when you feel like you need it.

5. 2. Cleaning Your Kidneys

Everybody's organs age at different times and rates. When you grow older, you want to drink less and less water.

That means your kidneys functioning job gets harder. That is why we need to remember to drink water, even if we don't want to or desire it.

Healthy lifestyle literature recommends that you need to remember to drink a cup of water in the morning before you even have your breakfast.

It's also a good idea to drink water before lunch. It's even better to drink water before dinner, too. Let's drink water with happiness and treat your body right.

Kidneys clean your body and your blood. It is important take care your kidneys.

Well then how do we do it?

IMAGINE that you are walking down a corridor toward the most beautiful door you have ever seen. You open the door an IMAGINE that you walk into a nice, cozy, warm room. When you get there, you take off your clothing and you go to sit in a chair in the middle of the room.

Then, IMAGINE how warm, refreshing rain runs through your neck and back.

In your mind, you are washing your kidneys that way. ALL of the acids, sugars, and salts MELT.

You see the water is super dirty that was collected. Your dirty water is allowed to flow into a container located on the ground next to your right-hand side.

Your kidneys became cleaner and they started to shine rainbow colors.

Then again, you IMAGINE how warm, refreshing rain runs through your neck, back.

In your mind, you are washing your kidneys that way.

ALL of the acids, sugars, and salts MELT.

Again, you see that the water is dirty, but not as much so as the first time, that was collected.

Your dirty water is allowed to flow into a container located on the ground next to your right-hand side.

Your kidneys are now 2 times cleaner.

Again you IMAGINE how warm, refreshing rain runs through your neck and back.

Again in your mind, you are washing your kidneys.

You clean out your kidneys a third time. You see the water that was collected is not dirty. Your water is allowed to flow into a container located on the ground next to your right-hand side. Your kidneys are now very clean. Your clean kidneys are enlightened in all the colors of the rainbow.

After this procedure, you must sit calmly for 3 minutes.

In the morning, when you wake up, remember to pee in a container to see how clean your kidneys became. Two days after performing this exercise, your kidneys should be super clean.

This exercise you can also perform in the spring

and fall or when you feel the need.

5. 3. Cleaning Your Liver.

Having a healthy liver is very important to one's life. The program that I propose depends on your thoughts—if you are an optimist and believe it will work, it will and if you are a pessimist and believe it will not work, then it will not. It all depends on you and your thoughts.

The liver is the organ which is especially involved in metabolism. It plays a protective role in protecting the body from harmful environmental effects and pollutants.

So make every effort to ensure that the liver will be healthy.

We know that the power of thought is unique and powerful.

IMAGINE that you are walking down a corridor toward the most beautiful door you have ever seen. You open the door an IMAGINE that you walk into a nice, cozy, warm room. When you get there, you take off your clothing and you go to sit on a chair in the middle of the room.

IMAGINE that warm water flows through the right side of your body. You use that warm water inflow to wash your liver.

While you wash your liver, the water becomes dirty from the MELTED away sugars, salts, and all the other substances contaminating your liver. Gather the dirty water. This dirty water is allowed to flow into a container located on the ground next to your right-hand side. Your liver is enlightened with the colors of the rainbow.

Again IMAGINE that warm water flows through the right side of your body.

You use that warm water inflow to wash your liver. While you wash your liver, the water becomes dirty from the MELTED away sugars, salts, and all the other substances contaminating your liver.

This dirty water is allowed to flow into a container located on the ground next to your right-hand side. Your liver again is enlightened with the colors of the rainbow.

For the third time, IMAGINE that the warm water flows through your right side.

You use that warm water inflow to wash your liver. Gather the now clean water. This clean water is allowed to flow into a container located on the ground next to your right-hand side. Your liver is brilliantly enlightened with the colors of the rainbow.

Your liver should clean itself in two-three days.

Repeat this exercise in the spring and fall, or when you will feel the need to do so.

All of this together helps the entire body to regenerate, recover and rejuvenate.

6. Your eyes.

We all know how important it is to have healthy, beautiful, glowing eyes. You should love your eyes, take care of them because they are the most important sensory organs you possess.

Eyes gather the most information from the environment. Eyes help a person focus on their environment, provide knowledge of the world, and are almost essential to studying.

E. Hess found the correlation between pupil size and our well-being - when we are rested, the pupil is at its largest, and the opposite is true when we are tired: therefore, it is essential to relax the eyes before going to bed.

Scientist Nile Bernick proved that male and female pupils increase in size when they are looking at a person they are interested in as a potential partner.

The computer has become a major part of our lives--used at work, used at home, used to gather information, used to contact friends, and so on. Everyone knows that the computer is harmful to our eyes, but not much is known about how to protect one's vision, especially if you have a lot of work to do on the computer. Eyes also get tired from using smart phones, tablets, and other devices with lit screens.

Therefore, it is important to give your eyes a rest during breaks. Experts recommend taking rest breaks at least five times a day.

It is also very important to relax the eyes before sleeping, if you lie down with tired eyes, then they will not be rested when you get up in the morning.

6. 1. Exercise to relax your eyes.

Mandatory conditions for eye relaxation exercises are: comfortable posture, warm palms (obtained by rubbing your hands together), slow breathing.

Eye relaxation exercises are a necessity if you want to improve your vision.

They must performed every day, at least 5 to 6 times, if not more per day, to again feel your full visual acuity.

This exercise is a very simple and effective. Your eyes will always look healthy, glowing, charming.

Sit down straight and comfortable. Legs bent at the knees at an angle of ninety degrees.

Hands should be warm, rubbing the palms of your hands until you will feel that the hands are warm.

Cup your hands and cover the eyes with the palms. The eyes should be covered so that light does not get through but the cupping should keep the hands from actually contacting the eyes.

Short easy breaths should be taken in through your nose, with a long, deep exhalation from the mouth.

Do this for one or two minutes. Depending on how tired the eyes are. After this procedure, you must sit calmly for 1 minutes.

7. Breathing exercises for the stabilization of the nervous system.

Breathing improves blood circulation and removes nervous tension. It also relaxes the body, improves sleep, puts one in a great mood, and increases the overall tone of the body.

Reflexes are innate (unconditional) or acquired (conditional).

We all have innate reflexes. You know that warm air expands blood vessels and that cold weather constricts blood vessels. The essence of the exercise is to expand and collapse the blood vessels. In this way we activate the capillary work.

The brain accepts the imagination as reality.
Sit down comfortably. Relax. Imagine that you are outdoors and a refreshing breeze tousles your hair, caressing your face. Breathe calmly with a SMILE.

When you inhale, you will feel the cool air. When you exhale, you feel warm air. The eyes may be closed to make it easier to concentrate.

Do this exercise very slowly and quietly, with concentration, and with a smile on your face.

Inhale a long, deep azure blue sky through your nose and allow it to fill all your flesh. Pause. Exhale the warm white of the sun's rays through the nose. Exhaled air waves drift far away to infinity. Pause.
Repeat the exercise six times.

Inhale a long, deep refreshing morning breath through the lower part of the neck, fill the whole body on the scent. Pause.

Exhale a long, warm sunny summer weather through the lower part of the neck. Exhaled air waves drift far away to infinity. Pause.
Repeat the exercise six times.

Inhale a long, deep refreshing morning breath through the solar ring. It is after chest above the stomach, fill the whole body on the scent. Pause.

Exhale a long, warm sunny summer weather through the solar ring (solar plexus). Exhaled air waves drift far away to infinity. Pause.
Repeat the exercise six times.
Inhale a long, deep refreshing morning breath

through the palms, allow it to fill all your flesh. Pause.

Exhale a long, warm sunny summer weather through the palms. Exhaled air waves drift far away to infinity. Pause.
Repeat the exercise six times.

Inhale a long, deep refreshing morning breath through the soles of the feet, allow it to fill all your flesh. Pause.

Exhale a long, warm sunny summer weather through the soles of the feet. Exhaled air waves drift far away to infinity. Pause.
Repeat the exercise six times.

Inhale a long, deep refreshing morning breath in through your eyes, allow it to fill all your flesh. Pause.

Exhale a long, warm sunny summer weather through your eyes. Exhaled air waves drift far away to infinity. Pause.
Repeat the exercise six times.

You have 30 seconds to sit and do nothing after

completing the exercise allowing your body to accept what you have done.

Our body has four medical extremities - two hands and two feet. We can massage and activate the biologically active points in the palms and the soles of the feet in a variety of ways.

You can massage any part or organ of the body, except the brain and the heart, by massaging biological checkpoints on your hands or feet, which correspond to the area where the problem is and you can breathe through it. As an example: it can be the ears, knees, kidneys, wrist, and so on.

8. Facial massage

The first law of well-being and healthy complexion is to drink a glass of water every morning before breakfast. This will improve the metabolism and digestion, and therefore the color of the face!

If you want to look your freshest, once a week you should put on a face mask made from:
--a quarter of an avocado,
--a half teaspoon of honey, and
--a half teaspoon of apricot oil.

Apply mask to your face and neck for ten minutes and then wash off with warm water.

Acupressure is one of the oldest treatments used widely in the East.

Spot Facial massage helps to reduce facial wrinkles, improves blood circulation and stimulates the skin.

Spot facial massage relaxes the entire body's muscles, relieves tension and spasms, improves micro circulation, and smooths out fine lines. After returning from work your face reflects tiredness and a lack of rest. In order to put your best face forward, in the evening you must perform facial massage.

Begin by sitting straight up on a chair because sitting up straight enhances your breathing. Place your hands on your legs. Close your eyes and breathe deeply for a couple of minutes.

Then you rub your palms together, because the hands should be warm. Bend your arms at the elbows palms facing up. Stay in this posture for at least 30 seconds. You are allowing energy to recharges your hands.

Place one hand, palm down, under your chin at one side or the other of your face.

Take the other hand, also palm down, and tap it against the first hand, moving from one side to the other and back again.

Do this three times.

Keep your mouth agape while doing the patting or tapping. This exercise relaxes the facial muscles.

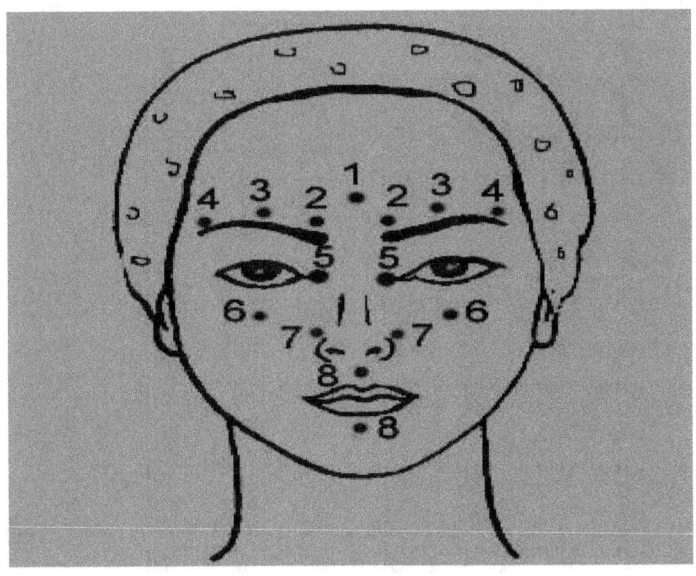

Point 1. This massage smooths out wrinkles on the forehead.

Take a fingertip and place it on point **1** a spot between the two eyes and slightly higher—the area where the third eye is located.

Move in a circle clockwise while counting: one, two, three, four, and five.
Move in a circle counterclockwise while counting: one, two, three, four, and five.

After finishing with the forehead circles, take the fingertips of both hands and gently tap all over the forehead in a random pattern for five seconds.
Point 2. Massaging them will help smooth out the wrinkles between the eyebrows.
Point 3. Massaging these points will help restore energy.
Point 4. Massaging these points will help improve the eyesight.

Place the tips of three fingers from each hand on the eyebrows at **Points 2, 3,** and **4.** Press easily while counting: one, two, three, four, and five.

Remove your fingers from the eyebrows and wait a couple of seconds.

Point 5. Massaging here will help improve the eyesight.

Place a finger near the inside corner of each eye on point **5** and against the side of the nose. Make tiny clockwise circles while counting: one, two, three, four, and five. Then make tiny counterclockwise circles while counting: one, two, three, four, and five.

Point 6. Massaging these will help keep the skin young and bright.

Take a fingertip from each hand and place it on **Point 6** on the bone underneath each eye and press easily while counting: one, two, three, four, and five.

Remove the fingertips from underneath each eye and wait for a couple of seconds.

Point 7. Massaging those helps smooth out wrinkles between the nose and lips.

Take a fingertip from each hand and place it on Point **7** against the side of the nostril and move in a clockwise circle while counting: one, two, three, four, and five.

Then move in a counterclockwise circles while counting: one, two, three, four, and five.

Point 8. Massaging them helps smooth out wrinkles around the lips

Take a fingertip from each hand and place one on the Point **8** in the center of the upper lip and the other just below the lower lip in the center. Make clockwise circles while counting: one, two, three, four, and five. Then make counterclockwise circles while counting: one, two, three, four, and five.

After finishing with the lips, take the fingertips of both hands and gently tap all over the forehead in a random pattern for five seconds.

Again, rub the palms of your hands together until the hands are warm and bend the arms with the palms up and facing outward to gather energy.

Then take your right and left hands. And hold

them from between a quarter of an inch to a full inch away from the side of your face.

The index finger of each hand should be next to but not covering the ear. Hold until you will feel warmth between the hands and your face.

Then make a counterclockwise circle while counting: one, two, three, four, and five. You will probably not be

The right hand should wind up at least over the forehead while the left hand winds up over the mouth area. Then imagine that you are collecting wrinkles and throwing them to the side.

Go back to the starting point and keep making a counterclockwise circle around your face without touching it. This time go smaller in scale with one hand at the top of the nose and one at the bottom of the nose.

At that point, make a grabbing motion with your hands and imagine that you are grabbing any wrinkles and imperfections you have and throwing them away. Do this a total of three times.

Next, place both hands alongside of the neck with the middle finger of each hand pointing toward the earlobe. Begin a counterclockwise circle with your right hand winding up under your chin and your left hand across the top of the chest. Make a grabbing motion with your hands gathering all the wrinkles and imperfections and discarding them.

Do this a total of three times with the counterclockwise circles becoming smaller with each pass. Never touch yourself with either hand and when you have gone as far as you can without getting your hands crossed make a grabbing motion and gather all wrinkles and imperfections in your hand and discard the This will lead to a lessening, if not disappearance, of wrinkles and an improvement in the quality of the skin itself.

9. Massage only for men

One exercise, specifically designed for men, is massaging the testicles. Every morning and every evening, a man should massage his testicles.

There is no specific manner or amount of time for this, although more is better than less.
This will help the strength of a man's bones, the strength of his erection, the healthiness of his skin, and will lessen the graying of his hair.